Living With...

# Obesity

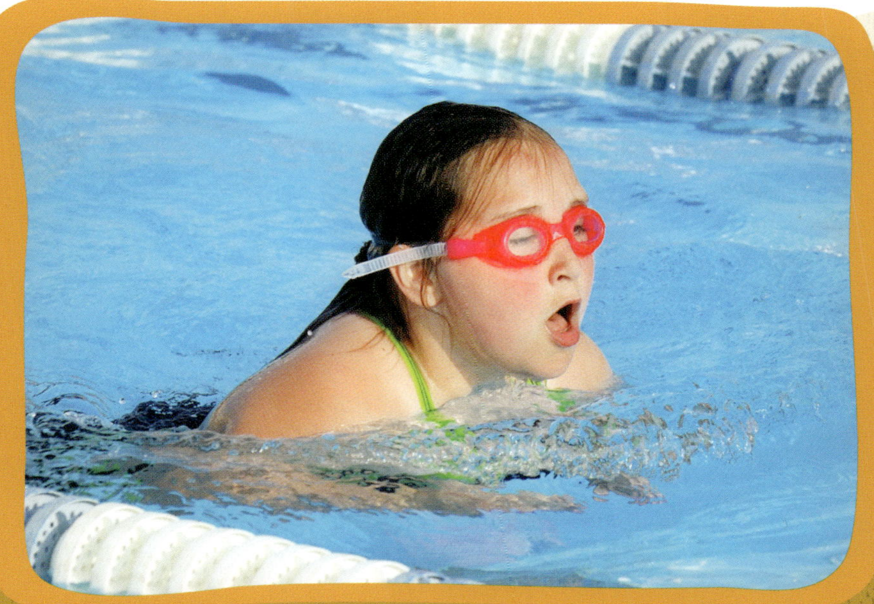

Nancy Dickmann

Consultant: Marjorie Hogan, MD

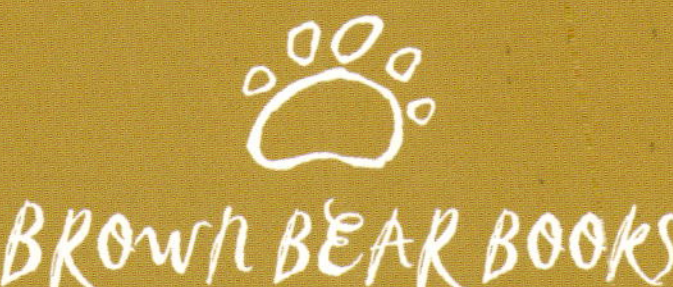

Published by Brown Bear Books Ltd
4877 N. Circulo Bujia
Tucson, AZ 85718
USA

and

Studio G14, Regent Studios,
1 Thane Villas, London N7 7PH, UK



ISBN 978-1-78121-806-8 (library bound)
ISBN 978-1-78121-812-9 (paperback)



Library of Congress Cataloging-in-Publication Data available on request

Text: Nancy Dickmann
Consultant: Marjorie Hogan, MD, Professor of Pediatrics, University of Minnesota, Retired staff pediatrician, Hennepin Healthcare
Design Manager: Keith Davis
Children's Publisher: Anne O'Daly

Manufactured in the United States of America
CPSIA compliance information: Batch#AG/5651

**Picture Credits**
The photographs in this book are used by permission and through the courtesy of:

Front Cover: Shutterstock: Kwanchai.c;
Interior: iStock: FatCamera 6-7, 18, mmg1design 22t, Monkey Business Images 12-13 SolStock 22b; Shutterstock: Africa Studio 8-9, Thomas Koch 4-5, margouillat photo 16-17, Monkey Business Images 6, 14-15, Motion Films 8, Olga Nayashkova 12, New Africa 20-21, Andrey Popov 10, Purdue9394 18-19, siam. pukkato 20, Red Stock 4, Syda Productions 14, Wavebreakmedia 16

All other artwork and photography
© Brown Bear Books.

t-top, r-right, l-left, c-center, b-bottom

Brown Bear Books has made every attempt to contact the copyright holder. If you have any information about omissions please contact: licensing@brownbearbooks.co.uk

**Websites**
The website addresses in this book were valid at the time of going to press. However, it is possible that contents or addresses may change following publication of this book. No responsibility for any such changes can be accepted by the author or the publisher. Readers should be supervised when they access the Internet.

Words in **bold** appear in the Words to Know on page 23.

# Contents

# What Is Obesity?

People come in all shapes and sizes. Some are tall. Others are short. Some have big feet. Others have long arms. These differences help make us who we are. They don't affect your health.

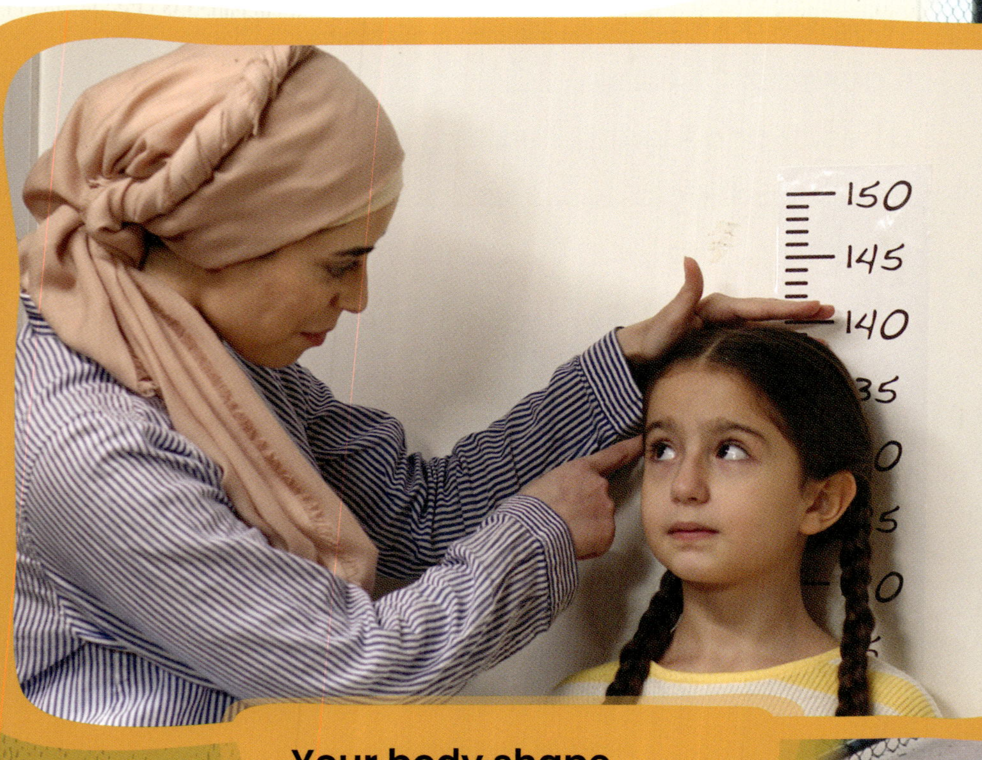


Your body shape changes as you grow.

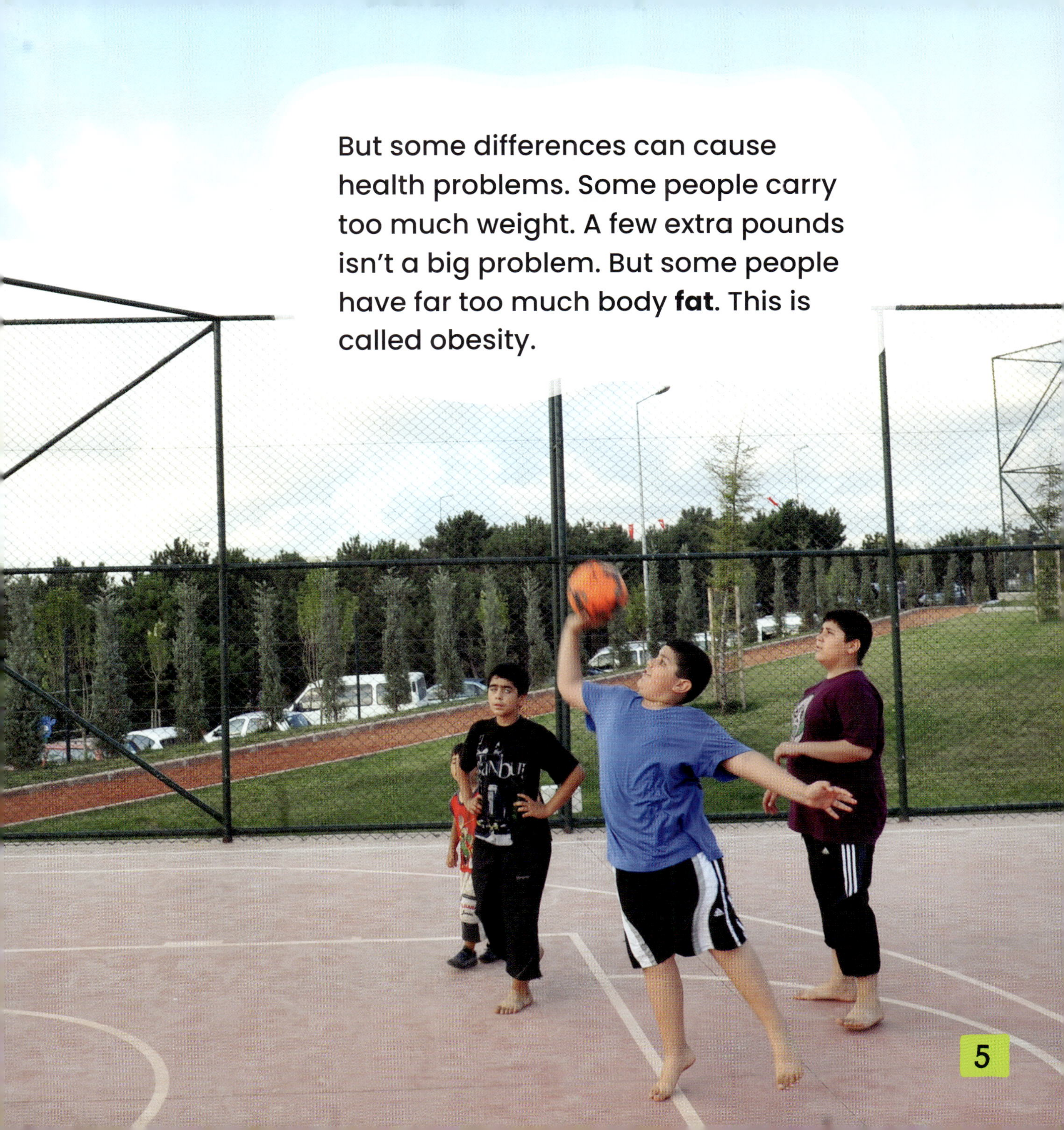

But some differences can cause health problems. Some people carry too much weight. A few extra pounds isn't a big problem. But some people have far too much body **fat**. This is called obesity.

# Measuring Obesity

Doctors often use a measurement called **BMI**. This stands for body mass index. They measure your weight. They measure your height. They use math to compare them. This gives them your BMI.

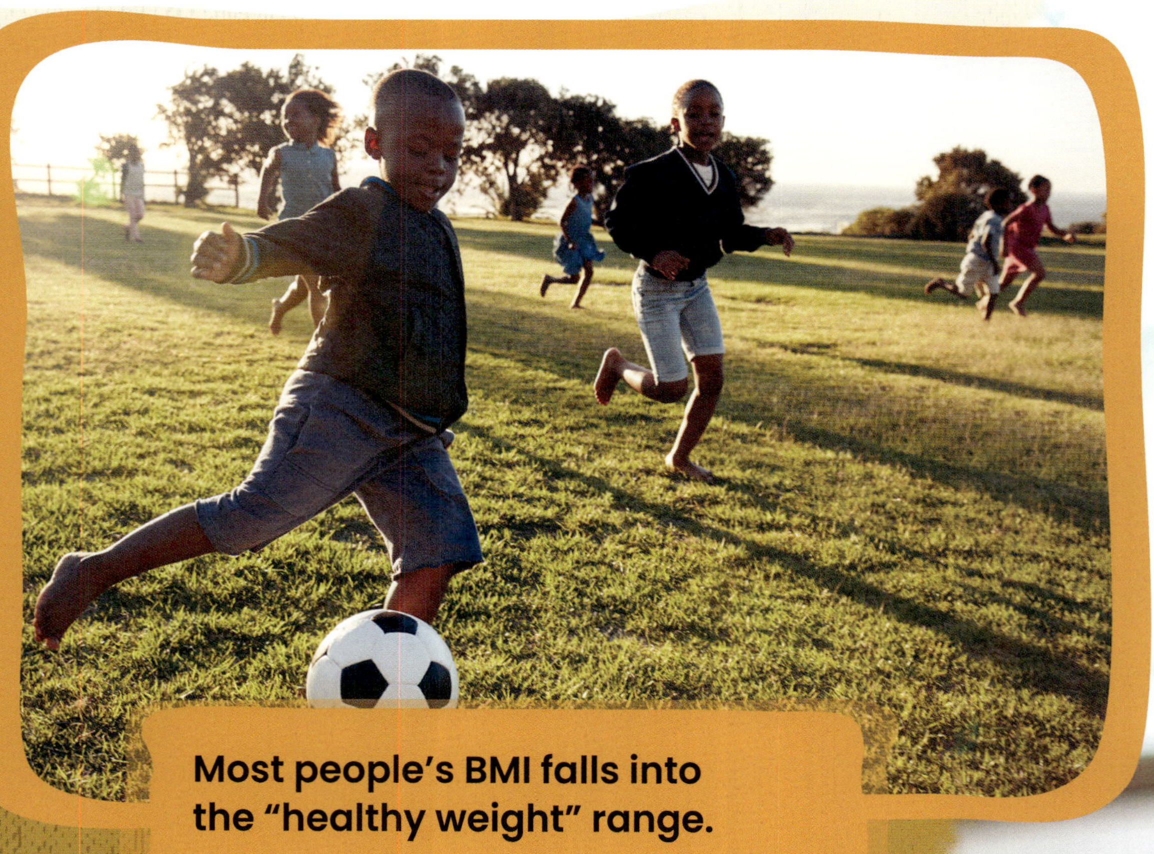

**Most people's BMI falls into the "healthy weight" range.**

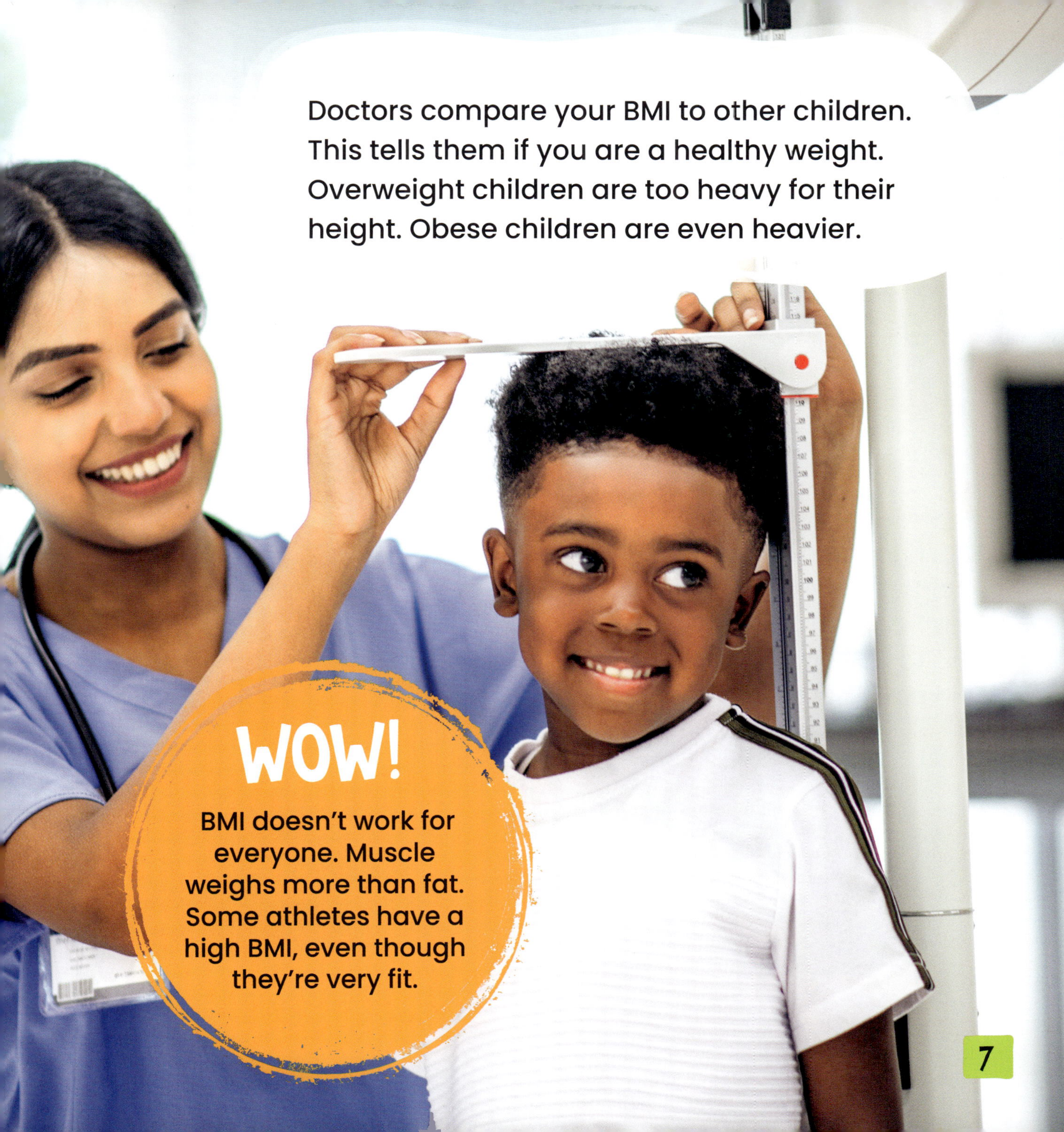

Doctors compare your BMI to other children. This tells them if you are a healthy weight. Overweight children are too heavy for their height. Obese children are even heavier.

## WOW!

BMI doesn't work for everyone. Muscle weighs more than fat. Some athletes have a high BMI, even though they're very fit.

# What's the Problem?

Being obese can make you feel tired. It makes physical activity harder. It often makes you sweat more. It can make you get out of breath.

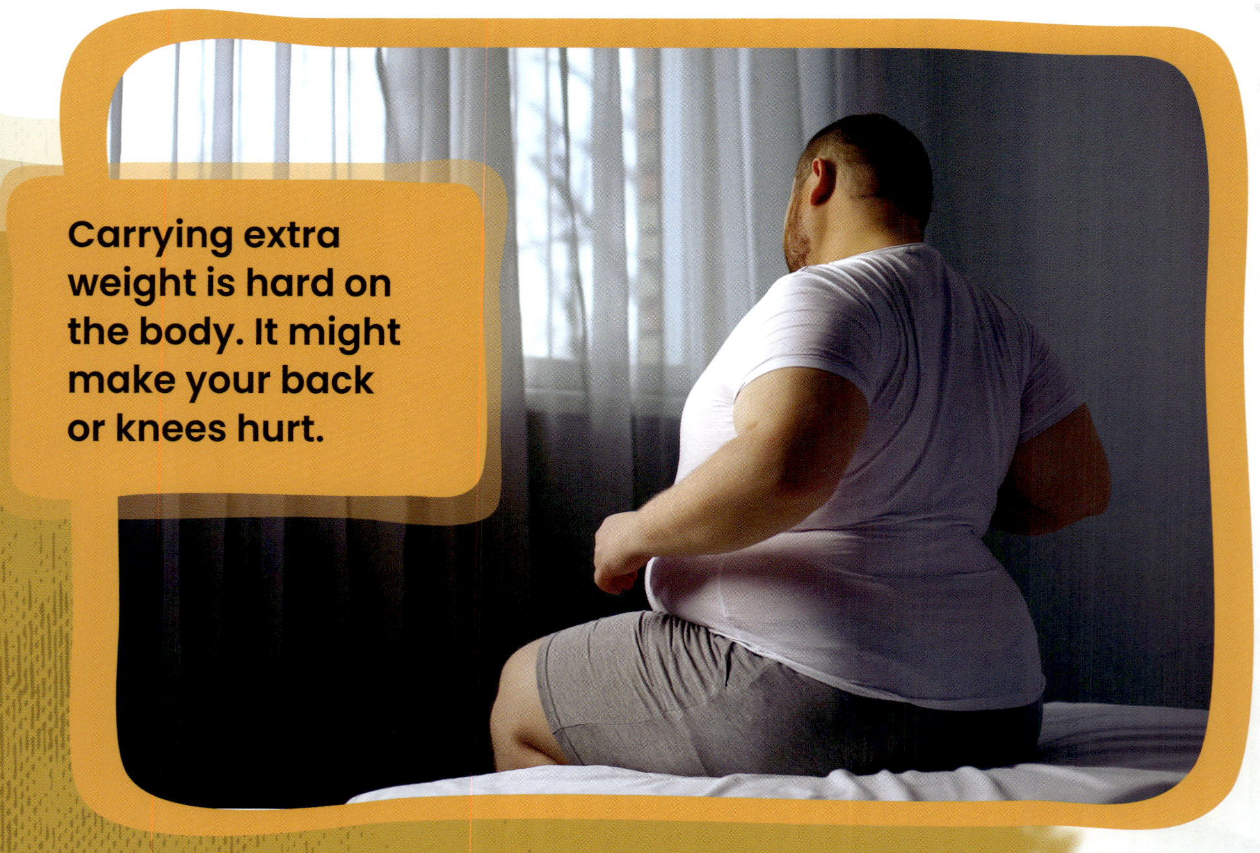

**Carrying extra weight is hard on the body. It might make your back or knees hurt.**

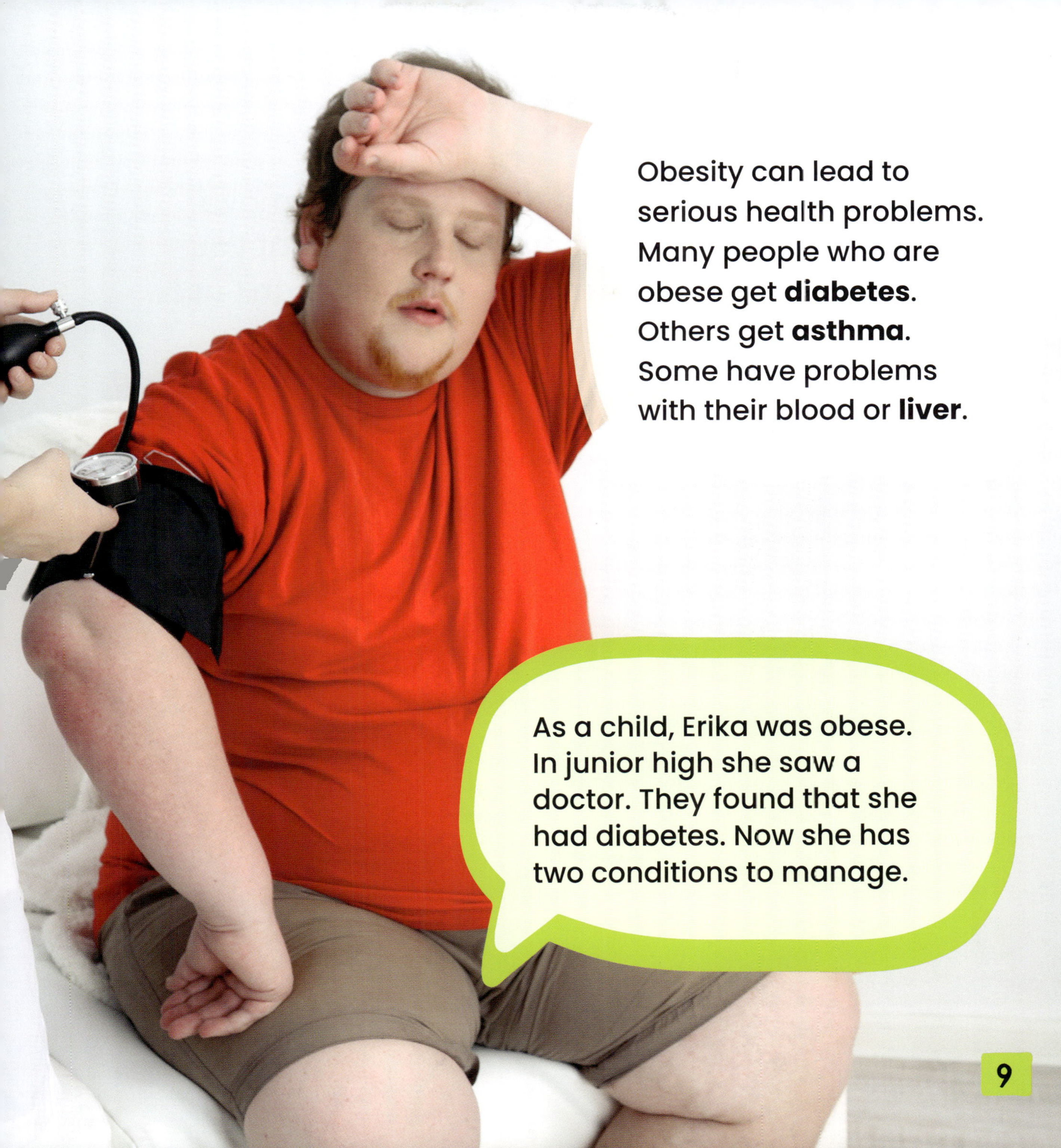

Obesity can lead to serious health problems. Many people who are obese get **diabetes**. Others get **asthma**. Some have problems with their blood or **liver**.

As a child, Erika was obese. In junior high she saw a doctor. They found that she had diabetes. Now she has two conditions to manage.

# How it Works

Food is **fuel** for your body. You need it to move and grow. Your body uses up most of what you eat. But if you eat too much, your body can't use it all. It gets stored as fat.

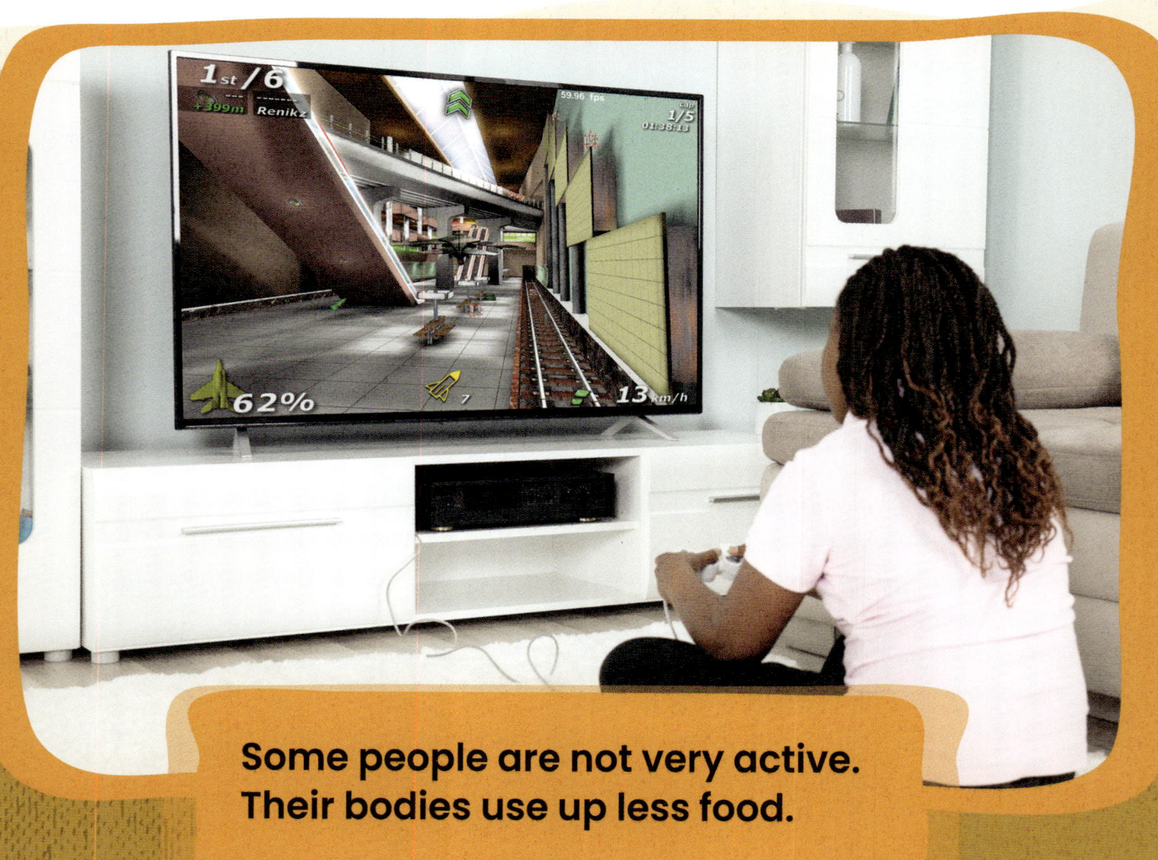


**Some people are not very active. Their bodies use up less food.**

You eat too much food.

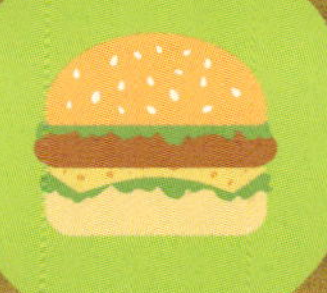

Your body uses the energy in the food.

Some helps keep your body working.

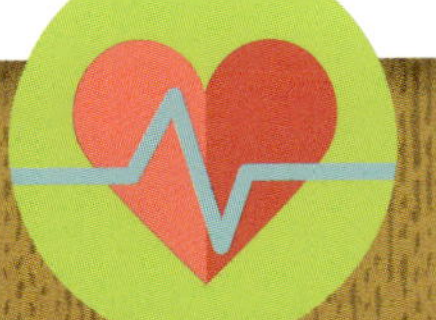

Some gets used up when you're active.

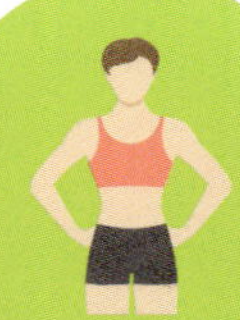

Some doesn't get used. It is extra.

Your body turns the extra food into fat. It stores it in case it is needed for energy later.

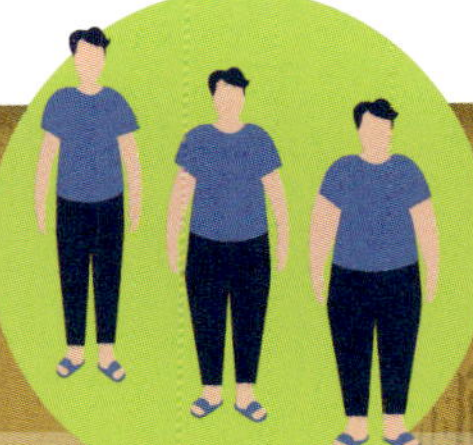

# Causes of Obesity

Obesity has two main causes. One is eating too much. The other is moving too little. The body can't use up all the food you eat. It stores it as fat. Over time, this fat builds up.

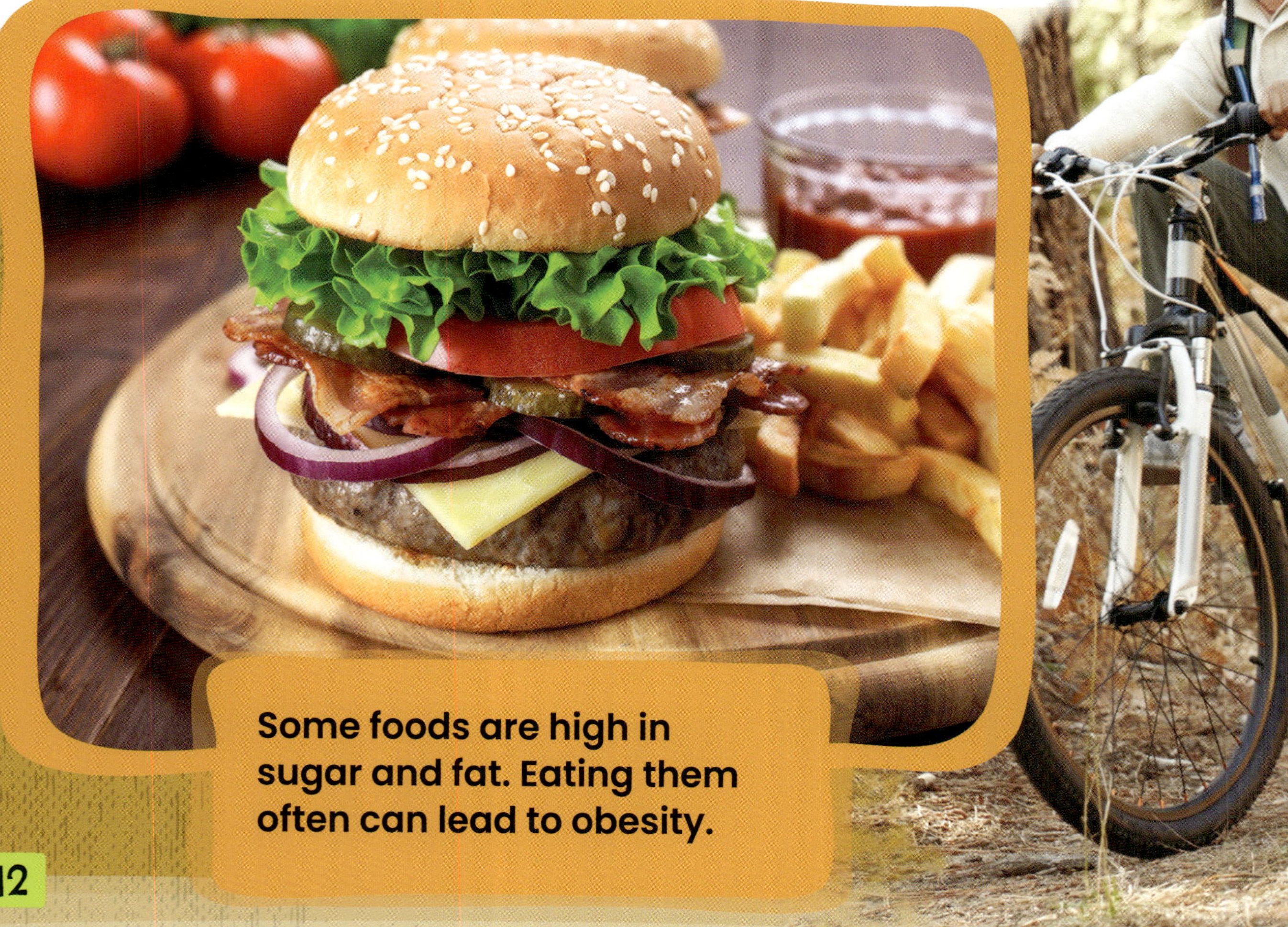

Some foods are high in sugar and fat. Eating them often can lead to obesity.

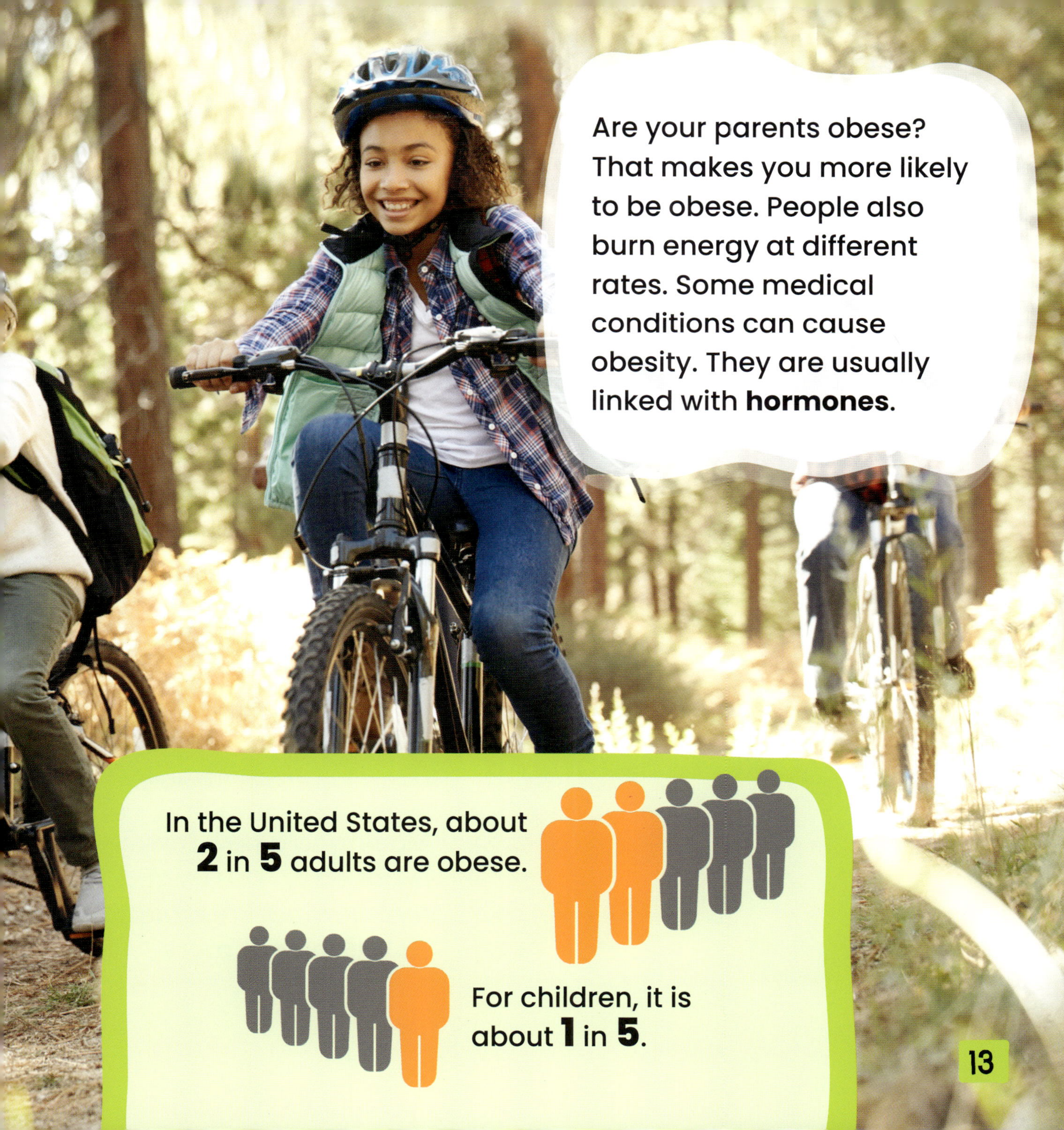

Are your parents obese? That makes you more likely to be obese. People also burn energy at different rates. Some medical conditions can cause obesity. They are usually linked with **hormones.**

In the United States, about **2** in **5** adults are obese.

For children, it is about **1** in **5**.

# Obesity and Mental Health

Mental health can also be a cause. Some people eat more when they are sad or upset. They choose foods that feel comforting. These are often high in sugar or fat.

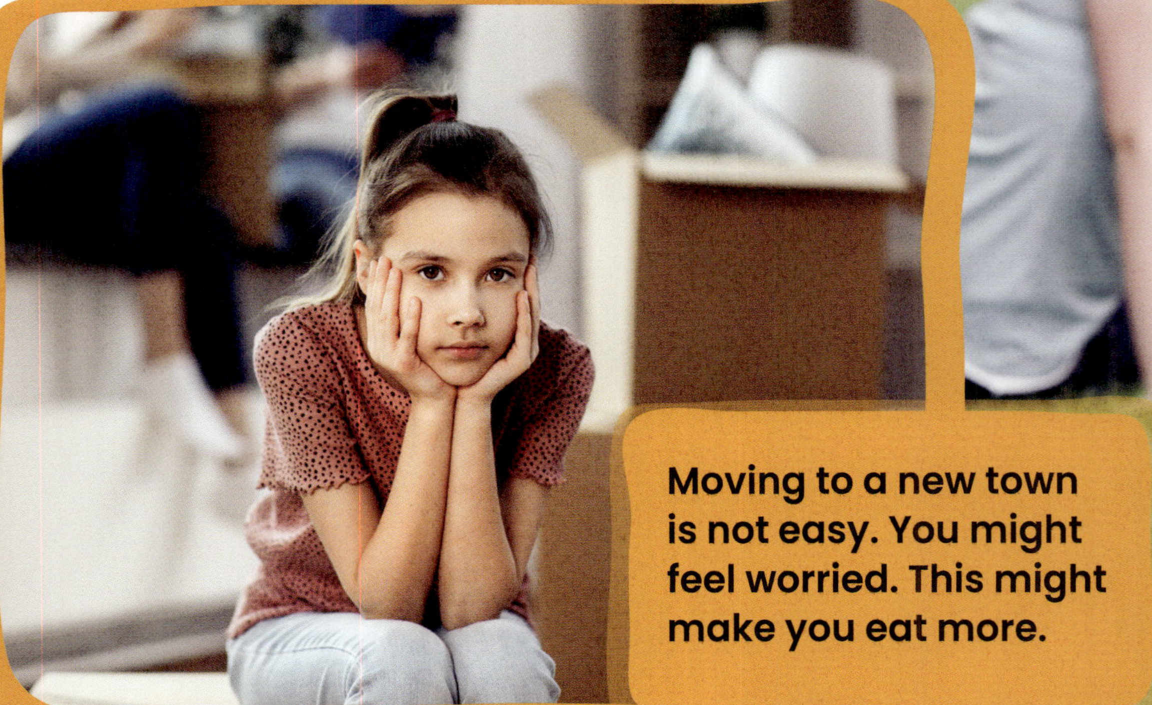

**Moving to a new town is not easy. You might feel worried. This might make you eat more.**

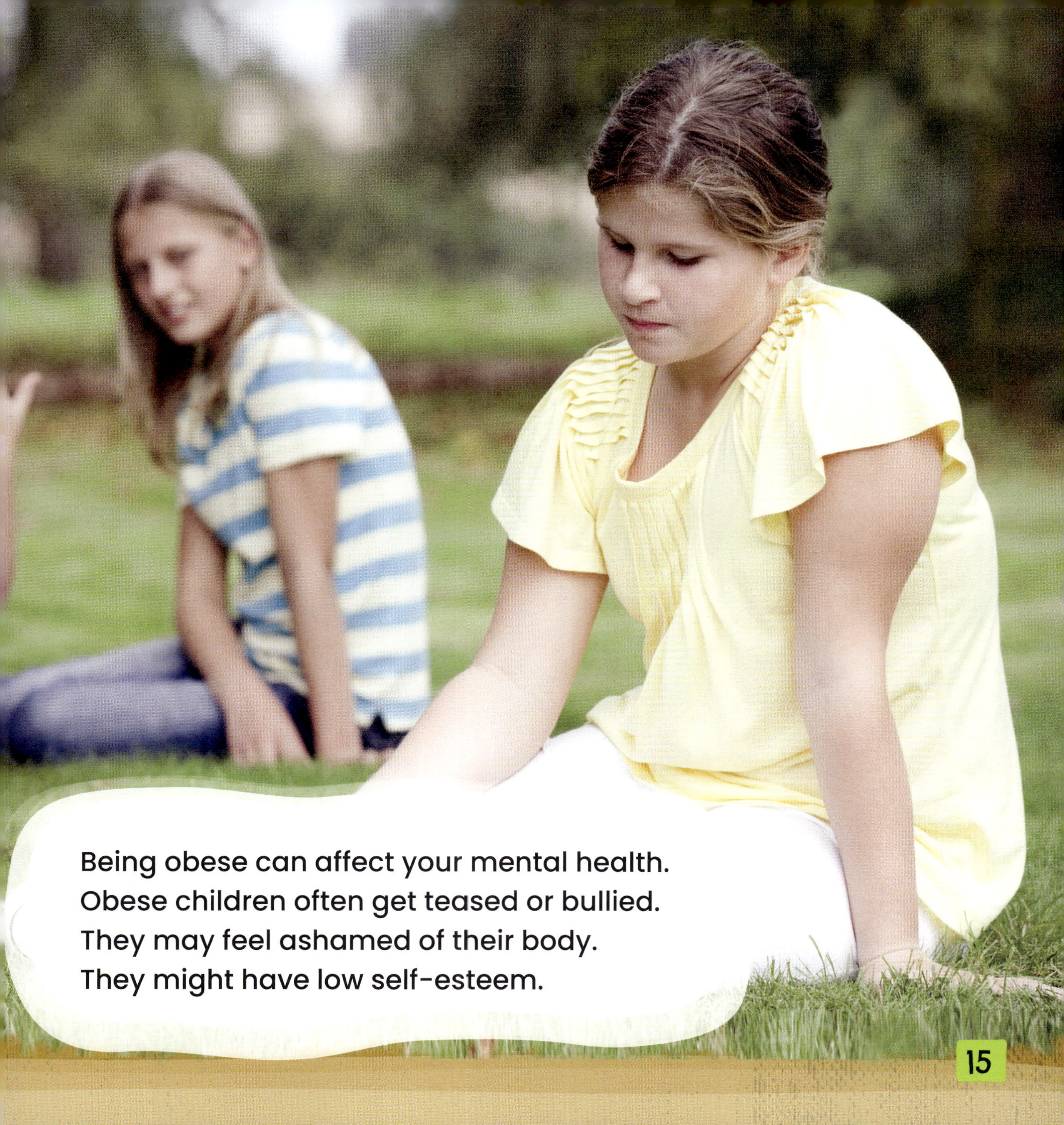

Being obese can affect your mental health. Obese children often get teased or bullied. They may feel ashamed of their body. They might have low self-esteem.

# Healthy Eating

You can treat obesity by getting back to a healthy weight. To lose weight, you eat less than your body uses. Your body needs to find more fuel. So it starts to burn stored fat.

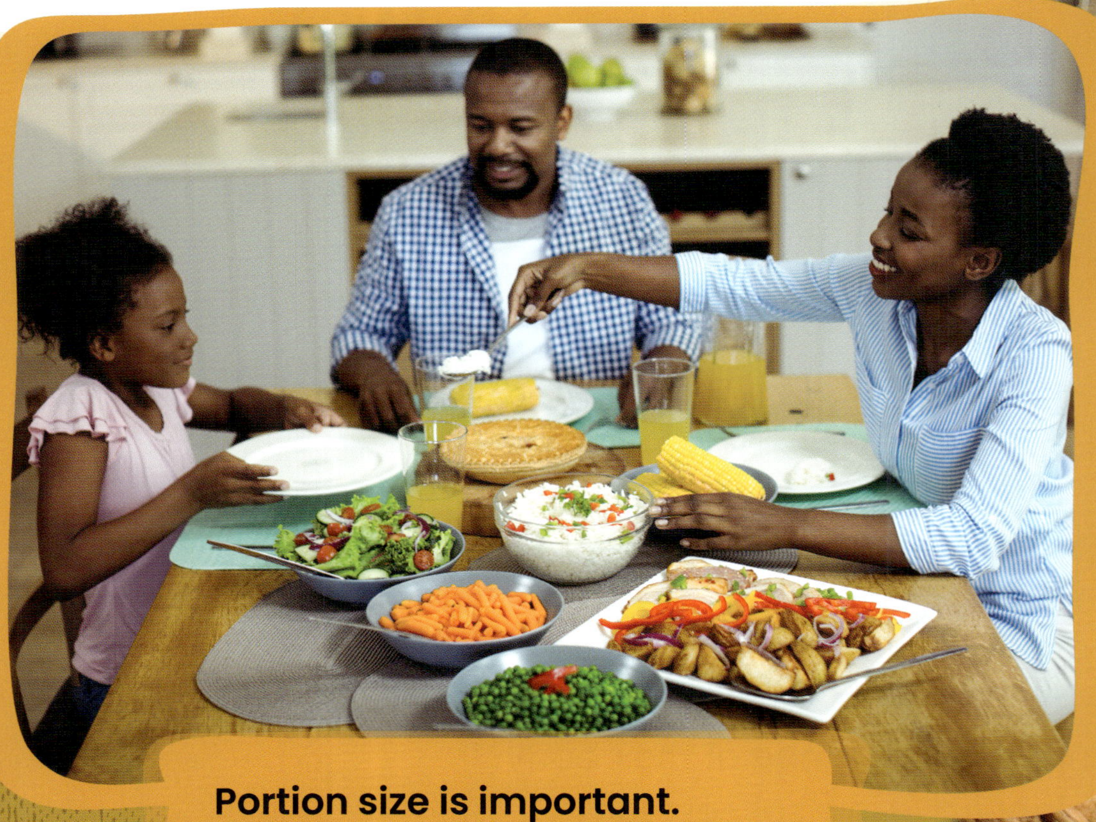

**Portion size is important. Eating smaller meals will help.**

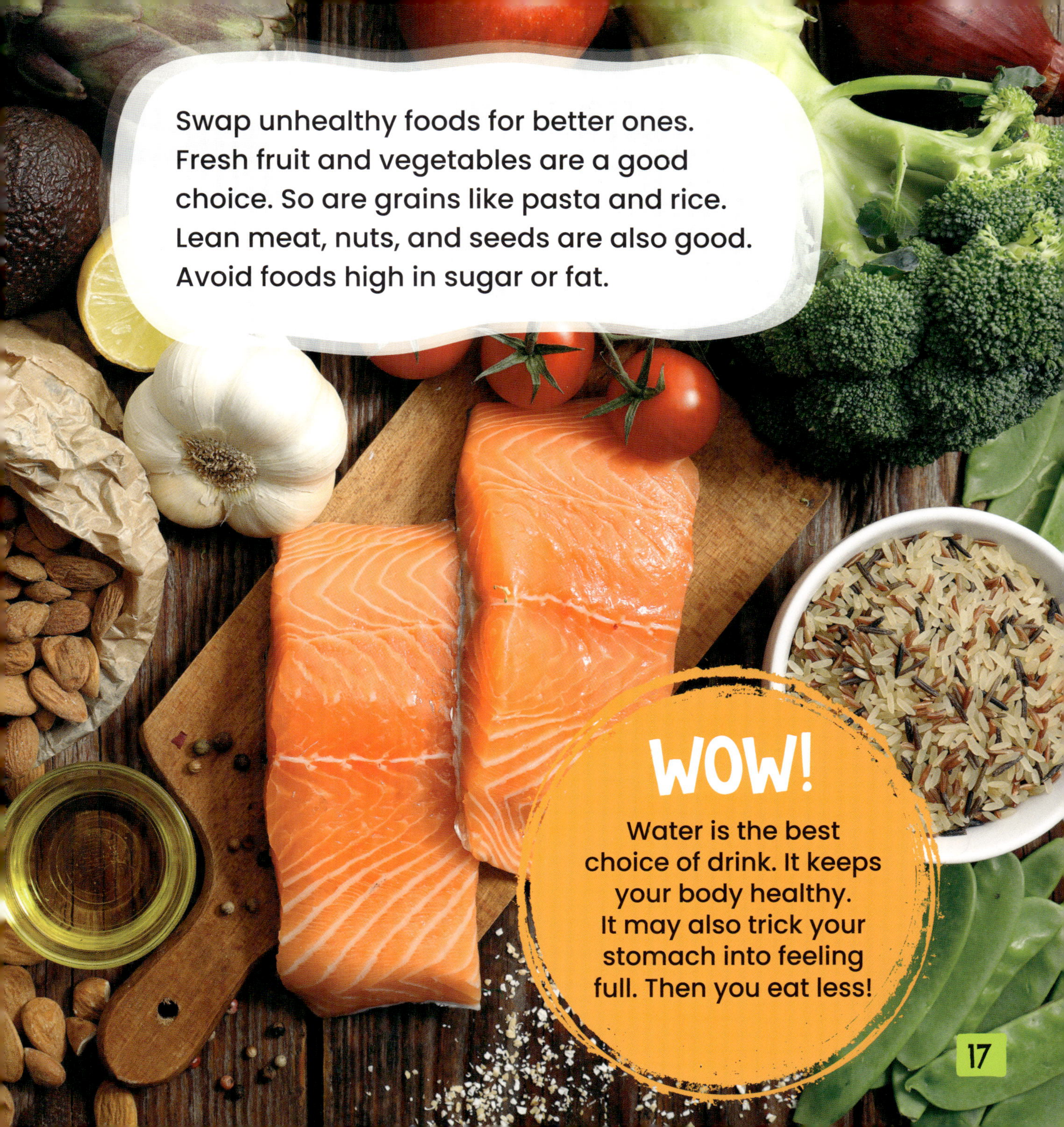

Swap unhealthy foods for better ones. Fresh fruit and vegetables are a good choice. So are grains like pasta and rice. Lean meat, nuts, and seeds are also good. Avoid foods high in sugar or fat.

## WOW!

Water is the best choice of drink. It keeps your body healthy. It may also trick your stomach into feeling full. Then you eat less!

# Staying Active

Eating less is only part of the solution. Staying active is also important. The more you move, the more fuel your body burns. It's fine to start small. How about going on a daily walk?

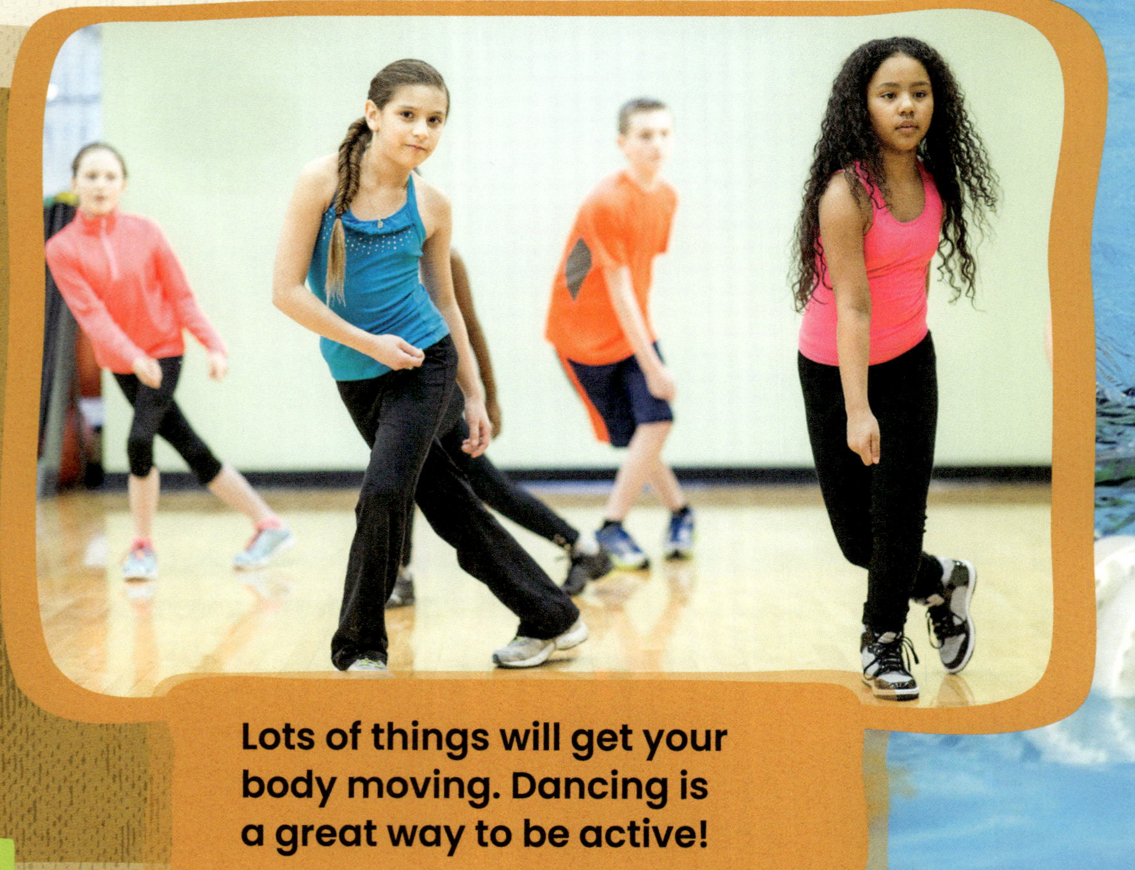

**Lots of things will get your body moving. Dancing is a great way to be active!**

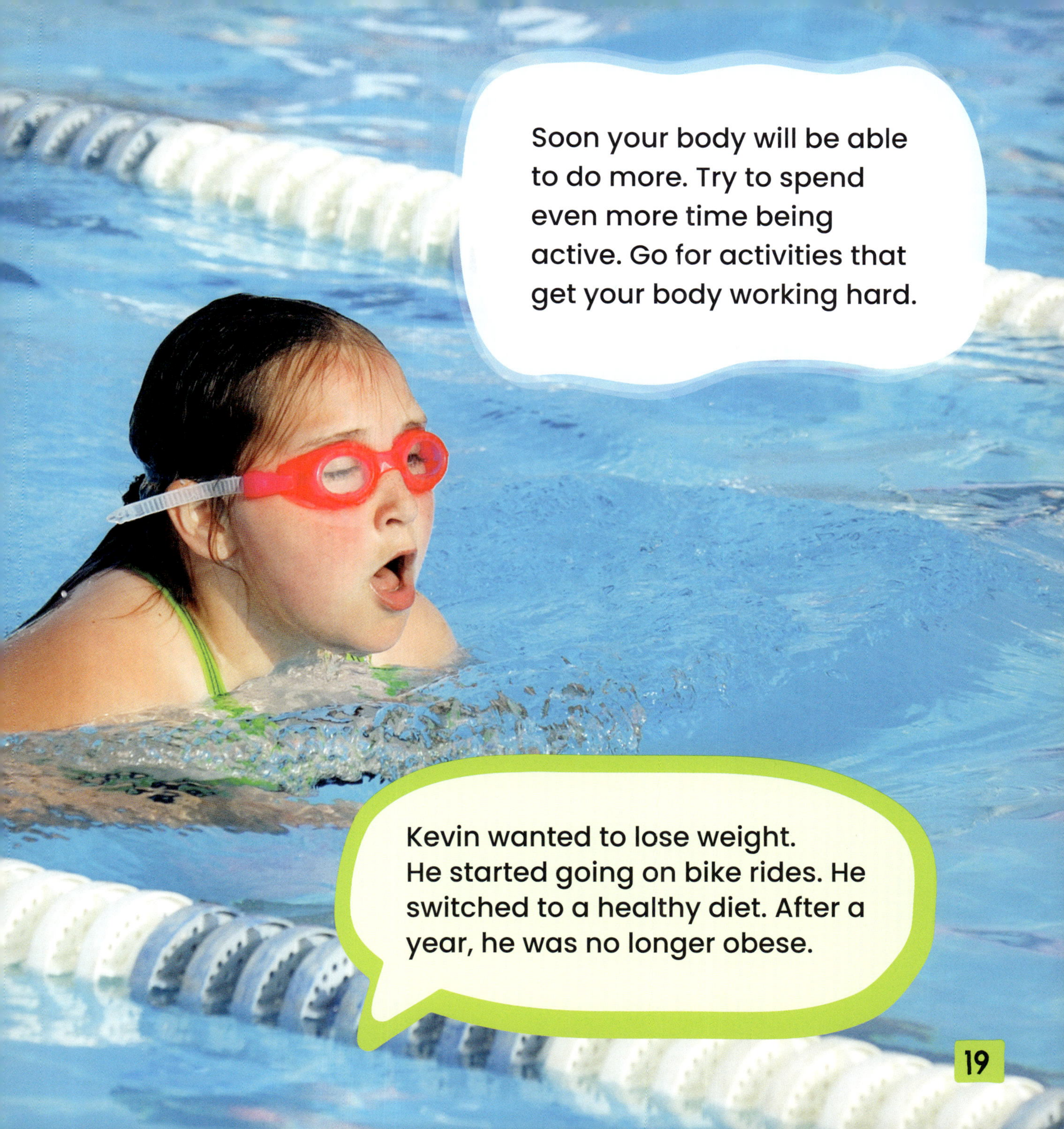

Soon your body will be able to do more. Try to spend even more time being active. Go for activities that get your body working hard.

Kevin wanted to lose weight. He started going on bike rides. He switched to a healthy diet. After a year, he was no longer obese.

# Other Treatments

Obesity can be reversed. But it may not feel easy! Losing weight takes time. It means sticking to your new routine. Medicines help some people. A doctor will decide if they're right for you.

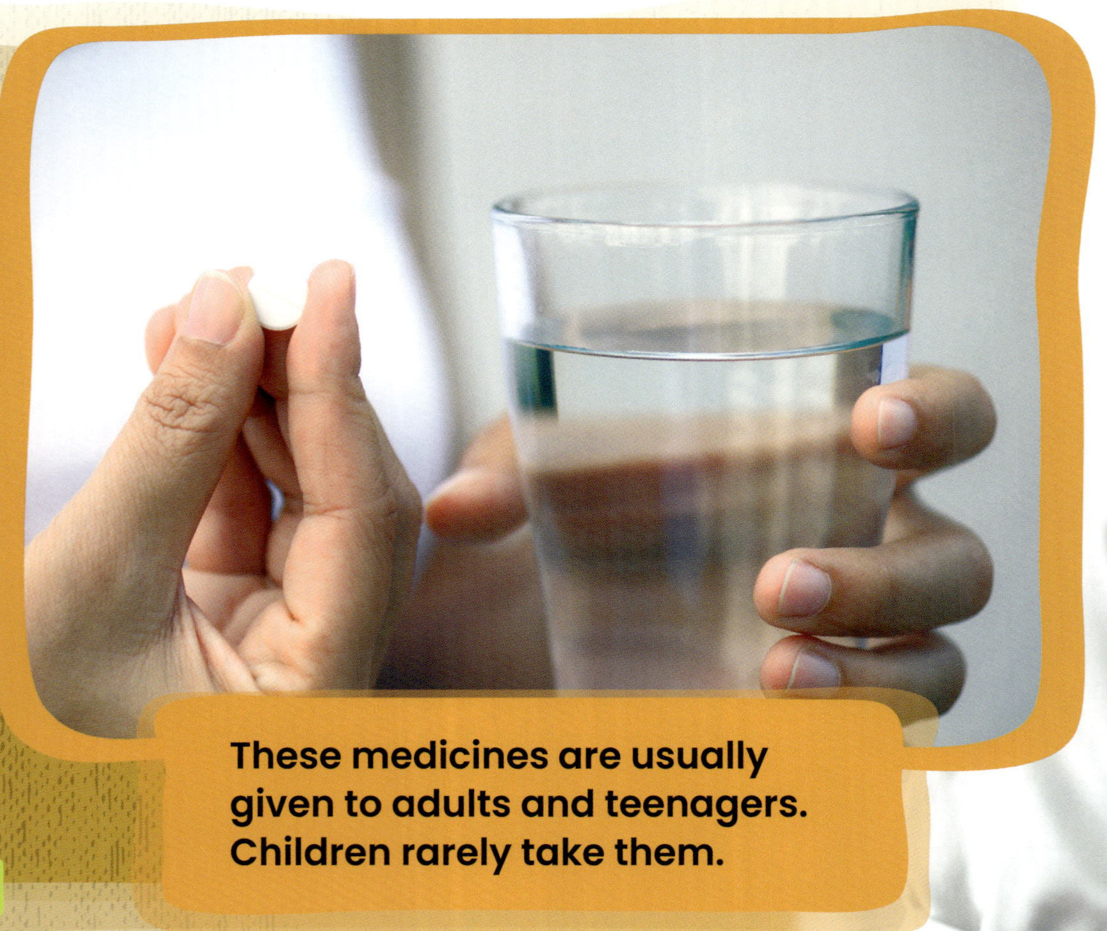

**These medicines are usually given to adults and teenagers. Children rarely take them.**

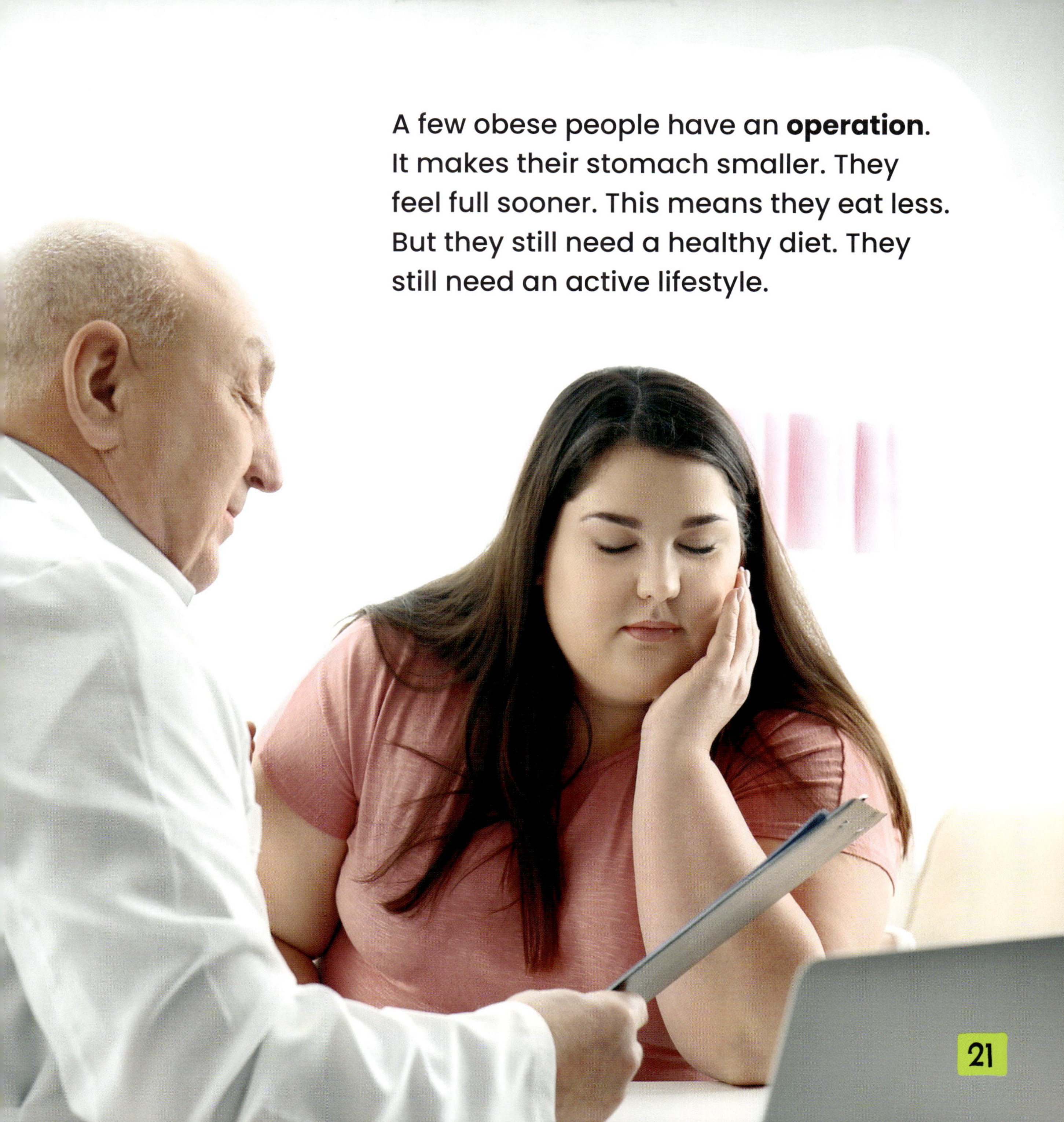

A few obese people have an **operation**. It makes their stomach smaller. They feel full sooner. This means they eat less. But they still need a healthy diet. They still need an active lifestyle.

# Activity

A healthy lifestyle is not just for people with obesity. It's important for everyone!

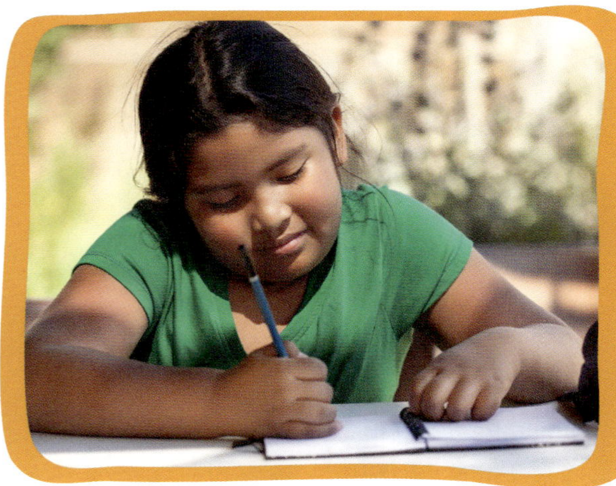

Keep a food diary for a week. Write down what you eat. How healthy is your diet? Could you swap out any fatty or sugary foods for healthier ones?

Keep an activity diary, too. Write down how long you're active. Don't forget things like walking to school or doing the vacuuming! Are you doing at least an hour each day?

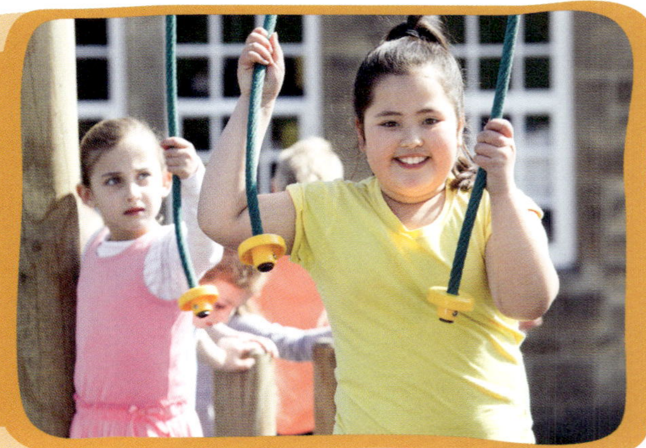

# Words to Know

**asthma** a medical condition that sometimes makes it hard to breathe

**BMI** a math formula that compares your weight to your height

**diabetes** a medical condition where the body can't easily break down sugar

**fat** a substance in some foods. It can build up in the body when you eat too much

**fuel** something that is burned to release energy

**hormones** chemicals that tell the body what to do

**liver** an organ in the body that helps break down the food you eat

**operation** when doctors cut into the body to fix something inside

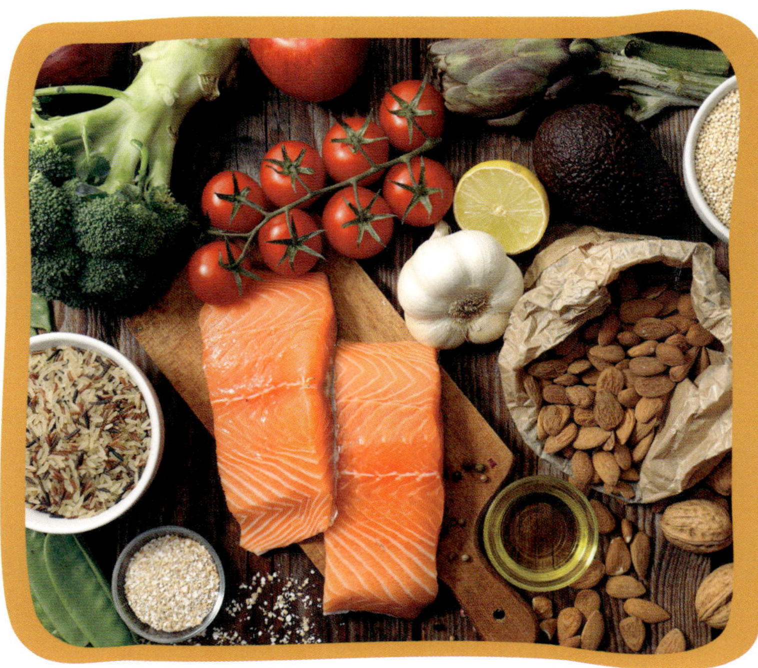

# Find out More

## Websites

dkfindout.com/us/human-body/keeping-healthy/

kidshealth.org/en/teens/obesity-overweight.html?ref=search

myplate.gov/life-stages/kids

## Books

**Healthy Body Image**
Martha E. H. Rustad,
Capstone, 2021

**Healthy Eating Habits**
Beth Bence Reinke,
Lerner Publications, 2019

**Staying Healthy**
Ashley Richardson,
Pebble Emerge, 2022

## Index